The Institute of Biology's
Studies in Biology

Medical Mycology

Mary P. English
D.Sc.

Consultant Mycologist, Bristol
Royal Infirmary and Research Fellow
in Mycology, Department of Botany,
University of Bristol

Edward Arnold

First published 1980
by Edward Arnold (Publishers) Limited
41 Bedford Square, London WC1 3DQ

British Library Cataloguing in Publication Data
English, Mary P
   Medical mycology. – (Institute of Biology.
   Studies in biology; no. 119   ISSN 0537-9024).
   1.   Medical mycology
   I.   Title   II.   Series
   616.9'69   RC117

ISBN 0-7131-2795-3

Printed and bound in Great Britain at
The Camelot Press Ltd, Southampton

General Preface to the Series

Because it is no longer possible for one textbook to cover the whole field of biology while remaining sufficiently up to date, the Institute of Biology has sponsored this series so that teachers and students can learn about significant developments. The enthusiastic acceptance of 'Studies in Biology' shows that the books are providing authoritative views of biological topics.

The features of the series include the attention given to methods, the selected list of books for further reading and, wherever possible, suggestions for practical work.

Readers' comments will be welcomed by the Education Officer of the Institute.

1980   Institute of Biology
                                         41 Queen's Gate
                                         London SW7 5HU

Preface

In Britain and Western Europe fungal diseases are a nuisance rather than a major problem. Ringworm and thrush are widespread and some forms are on the increase but they do not present a threat to life, while the potentially fatal primary systemic mycoses such as coccidioidomycosis and histoplasmosis, and the crippling subcutaneous mycetomas, are virtually unknown. Largely for this reason medical mycology receives scant attention in the curricula of either medical students or medical laboratory technologists and, although students of mycology and microbiology are taught many applied aspects of their subjects, medical mycology is seldom included.

However, modern therapeutic methods using steroids and immunosuppressive drugs, together with transplant and other massive surgery, have resulted in an ever increasing number of cases of potentially fatal, secondary systemic mycoses due to opportunistic fungi. Clinicians and laboratory workers alike now need a better knowledge of fungi as agents of human disease to enable them to cope with the new situation, and it is hoped that this introductory account, which assumes no previous mycological knowledge, will help towards this end.

I am grateful to medical colleagues at the Bristol Royal Infirmary for permission to use their clinical photographs to illustrate this book.

Bristol, 1980   M. P. E.

Contents

1 The Nature of Fungi

Fungi are eukaryotic organisms, that is, the nuclear apparatus is well differentiated and a membrane separates the nucleus from the cytoplasm. They are therefore quite distinct from bacteria. They are classed with algae and protozoans in the Protista, but they differ fundamentally from algae in that they have no chlorophyll and so are unable to photosynthesize their own carbohydrates from CO_2. Thus they are, of necessity, obligate parasites or saprobes, dependent on living or dead organic matter for their supply of ready-made carbohydrates. Fungi are much larger than bacteria (their vegetative cells are 2–10 μm wide) and they are morphologically more complex, with the result that their classification and identification are based primarily on their appearance and only secondarily on the nutritional and biochemical differences that are of such importance in bacterial classification.

1.1 The vegetative phase

In most fungi the vegetative phase (Fig. 1–1a, b, f) consists of filaments, or **hyphae**, with numerous lateral branches which together form the **mycelium.** This mycelium grows in or over the substrate and its functions are to absorb nutrients, to bear the reproductive organs, and sometimes to provide a resting phase to tide the fungus over a period of unfavourable conditions. While the hyphae of the more primitive fungi consist of continuous tubes with no cross-walls, i.e. they are **aseptate**, those of the more advanced groups, including most of those of medical importance, have **septate** hyphae in which the tubes are partitioned by more or less frequent cross-walls.

Resting spores of various sorts (Fig. 1–1c, d) are a response to adverse environmental conditions. Additional septa may be laid down in the hyphae which then fragment into chains of **arthrospores**, or some cells swell and develop thick, protective walls, when they are known as **chlamydospores.**

Fungi may not always form hyphae; some consist of separate round or oval cells which grow by budding out similar cells from their periphery. These are the yeasts (Fig. 1–1e). Many yeasts, including some of those of medical importance, also have a mycelial phase.

1.2 Sexual and asexual reproduction and classification

Fungal spores may be produced sexually (i.e. following a reduction division) or asexually, the two types being quite distinct from one another morphologically. Should both the **perfect** (sexual) and the **imperfect** (asexual) state of a given fungus be known they will almost certainly have been discovered at different times and will have been given different names. Both these names are valid under the International Code of Botanical Nomenclature, but that of the perfect state takes precedence over that of the imperfect.

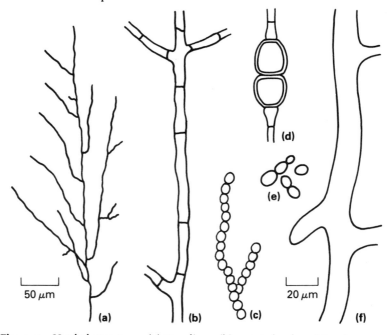

Fig. 1–1   Hyphal structures. (a) Mycelium; (b) septate hyphae; (c) arthrospores; (d) chlamydospores; (e) yeast cells and (f) aseptate hypha (Zygomycotina).

The classification of fungi is based primarily on their mode of sexual reproduction, i.e. their perfect state. Fungi of medical importance belong to the great subgroups **Zygomycotina**, **Ascomycotina** or **Basidiomycotina**. Sexual reproduction in the Zygomycotina is by fusion of the tips of two fertile hyphae with the formation between them of a single, large **zygospore**; in the Ascomycotina a sac or **ascus** contains eight sexually produced **ascospores**; and in the Basidiomycotina four **basidiospores** are borne on projections at the tip of a club-shaped **basidium**. Only if the perfect state is as yet undiscovered is a fungus classified in a fourth group, the **Deuteromycotina** or **Fungi Imperfecti**, a 'dustbin' group from which it will be removed when its perfect state is found. However, in practice many perfect fungi, including those of medical importance, continue to be known by the more familiar names of their imperfect states.

The beginner in medical mycology should be aware of the existence of the perfect state and of the niceties of nomenclature and classification which ensue, but at this stage a deeper knowledge of the imperfect state only is necessary. No further consideration will, therefore, be given here to fungal sex and its consequences.

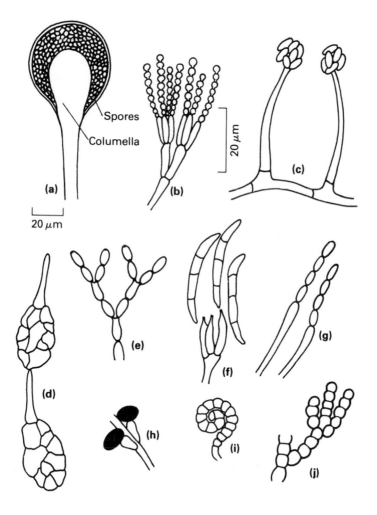

Fig. 1–2 Asexual spores. (a) Section of sporangium of *Absidia* sp.; (b) *Penicillium* sp.; (c) *Acremonium* sp.; (d) *Alternaria* sp.; (e) *Cladosporium* sp.; (f) *Fusarium* sp.; (g) *Geotrichum* sp.; (h) *Nigrospora* sp.; (i) *Helicosporium* sp. and (j) *Torula* sp.

1.3   Asexual spores

In those fungi with aseptate mycelium the asexual spores, or **sporangiospores**, are usually borne inside a closed **sporangium**, the wall of which breaks to liberate them (Fig. 1–2a). The sporangium, is carried on a stalk or **sporangiophore** which, in some fungi of medical importance, for instance *Absidia*, projects into the sporangium as the **columella**, persisting after the sporangium has burst.

In fungi with a septate mycelium the asexual spores, known as **conidia**, are not enclosed but are borne on conidiogenous hyphae either singly, in chains or in clusters (Fig. 1–2 b–j). If the ultimate cells of these hyphae abstrict the conidia from their open tips, as in the genera *Aspergillus*, *Penicillium* and *Fusarium*, they are known as **phialides**. The type and arrangement of the spore-bearing structures, and the shapes of the spores, are of infinite variety but are similar within each genus of fungi. They are of prime importance in identification.

Note

Though actinomycetes are now known to be bacteria, they were at one time thought to be fungi, and as a result of this confusion the diseases actinomycosis and nocardiosis, both caused by actinomycetes, are still included in text-books of medical mycology. They will not be discussed here. Neither will 'farmer's lung', an allergic condition caused by thermophilic actinomycetes growing in mouldy hay, which is often confused with allergic aspergillosis (see § 6.2).

2 The Pathogenic Status of Fungi

Few fungi are implicated as recognized human or animal pathogens, and the diseases they cause are of less importance than those due to bacteria and viruses. This is in marked contrast to the large numbers of fungal species that are responsible for plant diseases, often of the most devastating nature and extent. Again in contrast to plant pathogens, very few fungal species are obligate human or animal pathogens; most have a self-sufficient saprobic phase with a distinct ecological niche in the environment and are in no way dependent on the human host for their survival. But many fungi, such as species of *Aspergillus*, *Mucor* and *Cephalosporium*, which have been known as common saprobes since the early days of mycology, are now being implicated as occasional human pathogens following the introduction of new medical techniques which render the patient unnaturally susceptible to infection. Obviously therefore, a knowledge of the whole life cycle of potentially pathogenic fungi, including the saprobic phase, is essential to the understanding of the human **mycoses** (diseases due to fungi) and especially of their epidemiology.

In Table 1 human mycoses have been divided into five groups based primarily on the body tissue usually affected. Only the group of occasional pathogens and the unclassifiable disease candidiasis commonly affect a variety of tissues. The fungi causing the various diseases occasionally behave in an exceptional manner but this is unimportant for the purposes of the present study. Grouping the diseases in this way brings out clearly the increasing dependence of successive groups of fungi on the human host, and the way in which the site affected is related to the route by which the fungus enters the body. The diseases listed under each group are by no means exhaustive of the mycoses known, but are those which will be discussed in this book. They are representative of their groups and are described more fully in Chapters 6 and 7. For the record, some other important mycoses with their geographical distribution are listed in Table 2, though they will not be described further.

2.1 Primary infections, secondary infections and opportunistic fungi

Before embarking on a study of medical mycology, an understanding of these widely and often indiscriminately used terms is essential.

Primary infections are diseases occurring in otherwise healthy persons.

Table 1 Types of fungal disease with selected examples.

Type of disease	Causal fungi	Saprobic phase	Source of infection	Sites affected
Miscellaneous, due to occasional pathogens	Miscellaneous e.g. *Aspergillus* spp., *Acremonium* spp., *Schizophillum* sp.	Yes. Not recognized pathogens	Miscellaneous	Miscellaneous
Systemic mycoses Aspergillosis Cryptococcosis Coccidioidomycosis*	*Aspergillus fumigatus* *Cryptococcus neoformans* *Coccidioides immitis*	Yes. Soil, bird droppings, dead vegetable matter, etc. Recognized pathogens	Inhalation of spores from saprobic phase	Lungs primarily
Subcutaneous mycoses Mycetoma* Sporotrichosis*	Various moulds *Sporothrix schenckii*	Yes. Soil, plants, etc. Recognized pathogens	Wound by object contaminated by saprobic phase	Subcutaneous tissues
Dermatophytoses (ringworm, tinea)	Dermatophytes	No	Direct or indirect contact with infected host	Skin, hair and nails
Candidiasis (including thrush)	*Candida albicans*	Yes. Human commensal	Usually endogenous, occasionally contact	Many sites

* Not indigenous to Britain.

Table 2   Additional important mycoses.

Disease	Causal fungus	Geographic distribution	Notes
Systemic infections			
Histoplasmosis	Histoplasma capsulatum	North and South America; probably world wide	Intracellular parasite. Saprobic phase in bird and bat droppings
Blastomycosis	Blastomyces dermatitidis	North and South America; Africa	
Paracoccocioido- mycosis	Paracoccidioides brasiliensis	South America, Mexico	
Systemic phycomycosis	Absidia spp., etc.	Worldwide	
Subcutaneous infections			
African histoplasmosis	Histoplasma duboisii	Tropical Africa	
Chromomycosis	Phialophora spp.	Tropics and sub- tropics	
Subcutaneous phycomycosis	Basidiobolus spp.	Tropics	
Cutaneous infection			
Pityriasis versicolor	Malassezia furfur	Worldwide	Fungus a commensal of normal skin

Examples among the mycoses include the dermatophytoses, mycetoma, sporotrichosis and coccidioidomycosis.

Secondary infections are diseases which occur only in a host already weakened by some, usually unrelated, primary condition. Mycological examples include all the diseases due to the occasional pathogens, pulmonary aspergillosis and most cases of candidiasis; cryptococcosis can be a primary or a secondary infection. A normal, healthy person, even if he is in frequent contact with a fungus causing a secondary infection, runs little risk of contracting the disease because, in the unlikely event of the fungus penetrating the natural barriers of the skin, mucosae or healthy lung tissue, it is quickly dealt with by the body's normal immune defences.

Opportunistic fungi, or **opportunistic pathogens,** are fungi which have no need of a pathogenic phase for their own survival; their life cycle can be completed and their perpetuation ensured by means of the saprobic phase alone. But they are capable of pathogenicity should they encounter a human host in a suitably receptive condition. Strictly, all medically important fungi except the dermatophytes are opportunistic pathogens, for all except that group can flourish without at any time passing through a pathogenic phase. But a few, notably *Coccidioides immitis* and *Histoplasma capsulatum*, are so well adapted to a pathogenic role that they are omitted from consideration as opportunists. Opportunists, therefore, include all fungi classed as secondary pathogens, together with those causing the subcutaneous mycoses which must be introduced into the body through a wound.

2.2 Allergy and toxicity

Invasion of the tissues is not the only way in which fungi can induce disease in man. The airborne spores of a number of species may cause asthma, 'hay' fever and other respiratory diseases if inhaled by sensitive persons. Such allergic conditions will be discussed more fully in Chapter 9. Other species ranging in type from toadstools to moulds cause severe or fatal poisoning, either immediately or over a period of time, if they or their metabolic products are eaten. Chapter 10 is devoted to myco-toxicosis and mycetism.

3 The Saprobic Phase

Because all the fungi causing subcutaneous and systemic mycoses, allergy and toxicity are saprobes in the normal course of events (Table 1), those working with medical fungi must be familiar with the saprobic lives of their organisms.

3.1 Substrates

In general, fungi are better adapted to growth on vegetable than on animal substrates and this is also true of most potential human pathogens. Many are soil inhabitants; *Sporothrix schenckii* is found on the surfaces of plants, particularly of trees; coprophilous species such as *Cryptococcus neoformans* are usually found in the droppings of seed-eating birds such as pigeons and domestic fowls; and *Aspergillus fumigatus* is a ubiquitous agent of the decomposition and decay of almost any sort of dead vegetable matter.

3.2 Temperature

All potential human pathogens except those confined to the skin and its appendages are, of necessity, capable of growth at 37°C, but their optima may vary considerably. For instance, *Cryptococcus neoformans* prefers about 35° while *Aspergillus fumigatus* grows best at 45°, but both temperatures are much higher than those normally encountered away from the host. Temperatures far below the optimum reduce the growth rate, and therefore the competitive ability of a fungus. This problem is overcome by *A. fumigatus* which thrives in the heat generated during the decomposition of its vegetable substrate, for the temperature within a compost heap or bale of damp hay may easily rise to 45°. The temperature of the bird droppings favoured by coprophilous fungi could also rise during the early stages of degradation, but that of substrates inhabited by other fungi will depend on their geographic location and exposure to sunshine.

3.3 Moisture

Although the mycelium and spores of many fungi can survive prolonged periods of desiccation, for active growth the mycelium needs a moisture content in the substrate of at least 14–20%, a level which would not be uncommon in nature. For sporulation however – and it is by

means of their asexual spores that most saprobes effect their entry into the
human host – a much higher moisture content is necessary. Conidium
production may therefore be sporadic, occurring only after rain or heavy
dew.

3.4 Competition with other microorganisms

Any saprobe growing in the wild must face competition from other
microorganisms, and its success in the struggle will depend either on an
extremely favourable environment which allows it to grow so exuberantly
that it overwhelms competitors, or on especially difficult circumstances,
with one important constituent of which the fungus is better able to cope
than its competititors. In an environment in which nutrients, available
moisture, pH and temperature are all optimal for the fungus they are
likely to be favourable for many other organisms too, so that these may
gain the upper hand by sheer weight of numbers. So survival of the fungus
may well depend on an unusual ability to grow, if slowly, at some
physiological extreme, or to utilize some unusual nutrient which few
competitors can tolerate. Few organisms, for instance, can survive the
high temperatures enjoyed by *Aspergillus fumigatus* in a compost heap.
Coccidioides immitis also survives in the saprobic phase by avoiding
competition. Coccidioidomycosis occurs only in the South West U.S.A.,
Central America and northern South America. This is a semi-desert area
and the spores of *C. immitis* are adapted to survive the summer in the hot,
dry, saline and very sandy soil which few other microorganisms can
tolerate. It is impossible to find the fungus in adjacent areas of richer,
moist soils which can support competitors.

3.5 Geographical distribution

Enough has been said about the growth requirements of the saprobic
phases of pathogenic fungi to indicate that some mycoses at least will be
confined to limited geographic areas where those conditions can be met.
Coccidioidomycosis for the reasons just given, is one of the most clearly
demarcated of these diseases. *Cryptococcus neoformans* on the other hand, is
found wherever there are pigeon droppings, and cryptococcosis occurs
sporadically in many parts of the world. A number of different fungi can
cause the clinical condition known as mycetoma and it has been found
that each has a distinct climatic preference. Cases due to *Madurella
mycetomatis* for instance are found in tropical countries with a moderate
rainfall, but in places with a very high rainfall *Petriellidium boydii*
predominates.

3.6   Spore dispersal and entry into host

Spores produced in saprobic life are of paramount importance in the induction of the systemic and subcutaneous mycoses and in allergic conditions, and the way in which they are dispersed will determine the route by which they enter the body and hence the type of disease they cause. Fungal spores, both sexual and asexual, may be adapted for dispersal in various ways, some by air currents, some by rain or dew, some sticky spores become attached to insects, and elaborately shaped spores depend on running water for dispersal.

'Dry spores' are air dispersed. They have water-repellant walls and may remain airborne for long periods. The fungi producing them are among the most common laboratory contaminants, and include such well-known genera as *Aspergillus*, *Penicillium* and *Cladosporium* (Fig. 1–2). All fungi causing systemic mycoses have dry spores which enter the host by the respiratory route. Some dry-spored fungi also cause allergic conditions such as asthma and 'hay' fever (see Chapter 9).

'Wet spores' are dispersed by rain or dew and usually have hygroscopic surfaces. Many, when wet, have a coating of slime which helps them to stick to the substrate until germination begins. Subcutaneous mycoses are usually caused by wet-spored fungi which are inoculated into the host through a wound or in some similar way.

4 The Host in the Fungal Life Cycle

Table 1 shows how the fungi causing human disease differ from each other in their dependence on the living host. While the agents of the systemic and subcutaneous mycoses are fully capable of an independent life as saprobes, those causing dermatophytosis and candidiasis are, in their different ways, wholly dependent on their human substrate. This clearly has a considerable bearing on the epidemiology of the various types of mycosis, so we shall now consider the fungi from this point of view.

4.1 Fungi independent of the host

We have seen that the miscellaneous mycoses due to common saprobes and the subcutaneous and systemic mycoses are all caused by fungi which normally lead a blameless saprobic life. Although the habitats of some of them have yet to be discovered, there is no doubt that each has a regular ecological niche where it can grow successfully in competition with other saprobic microorganisms.

Most fungi show a preference for low temperatures, perhaps around 20°C, but human pathogens, except for skin pathogens, must be able to grow at the body temperature of the host, that is at 37°C. In theory, any fungus which can tolerate such temperatures is a potential pathogen and, in fact, more and more of those previously thought to be purely saprobic are now being incriminated as occasional human pathogens.

Whether they are frequently or only occasionally pathogenic, saprobic fungi are ill-adapted to the parasitic state in one important way; no means of cross-infection from host to host has been evolved. Each new infection must be contracted afresh from the saprobic phase and the parasitic state is a dead end in the life cycle of the fungus. Consequently, in the management of cases of systemic and subcutaneous mycoses, precautions against cross-infection are pointless. However, the fungi are so much a part of their environment that attempts to prevent the spread of infection by eliminating the saprobic phase are usually also doomed to failure. The diseases can only be prevented by ensuring that the fungi do not enter the body, which is often impractical or, while taking no action against the fungi, by raising the immune status of the potential host. Entry into the body can most easily be prevented in some subcutaneous mycoses, many cases of which could be avoided if agricultural workers in areas in which the diseases occur, **endemic areas**, had adequate protection for their feet and legs. Vaccination against mycoses is not at present practicable, but any step towards improving the general health of a patient is a step towards the prevention of systemic fungal infection.

4.2   Fungi dependent on the host

4.2.1   Total dependence: parasitism

The dermatophytoses, or ringworms, are caused by three closely related genera of fungi known as the **dermatophytes** all of which, when growing on a keratinized substrate in the saprobic phase digest it in a characteristic way. When attacking a hair these fungi penetrate under the cuticle and between the cells of the cortex by means of flattened, frond-like mycelium (Fig. 4–1a). Also columns of wide cells, the **perforating organs**, grow radially into the cortex forming deep pits (Fig. 4–1b). Around both fronds and perforating organs are wide zones of

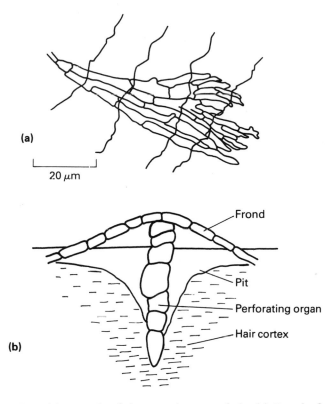

Fig. 4–1 Saprobic growth of dermatophytes on hair. (a) Frond of eroding mycelium beneath cuticle scales. (b) Radial penetration of hair shaft by a perforating organ.

keratinolysis, but the chemistry of the lytic action is at present disputed. This combined mechanical and lytic attack can destroy the hair in a few weeks (Fig. 4–2).

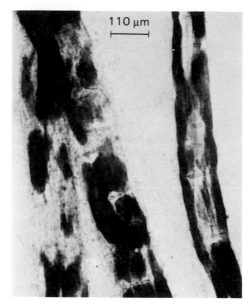

Fig. 4–2   Hairs on which a dermatophyte has been cultured for two weeks. In the unstained parts the keratinized tissue has been replaced by a mass of mycelium. Lactophenol-cotton blue.

Although all the dermatophytes are able to destroy isolated keratinized tissues by this process or slight modifications of it, most are, in fact, unable to survive as free-living saprobes in competition with other microorganisms and therefore can make no use of their capability. Of the common dermatophyte species thirteen are **anthropophilic**, that is, they are found only in human ringworm lesions and are entirely dependent on passage from human host to human host for the survival of their race. Twelve species are **zoophilic**, that is they are primarily dependent on an animal for survival, and although all can also cause ringworm in man, none can survive as a saprobe for more than a short while. Only three dermatophyte species are **geophilic**, that is, they are common soil saprobes, and human ringworm caused by these species is rare. Only these three, of all the pathogenic dermatophyte species, are in no way dependent on the living host for survival and these could justifiably be included in the group of occasional pathogens.

In addition to those geophilic dermatophytes which occasionally cause human ringworm, there are many other closely-related species which are entirely non-pathogenic, and there seems to have been a gradual evolution from these unspecialized saprobic forms to those which are now so specialized as to be obligate human pathogens. In the course of this evolution, although the fungi have retained their distinctive means of digesting keratinized materials as saprobes, many now no longer have the ability to reproduce sexually or even, in the case of some anthropophilic species, asexually. These changes are summarized in Table 3.

Table 3 Fertility in the dermatophytes and their saprobic allies.

Pathogenic status of fungus	Preferred habitat			Reproduction	
	Soil	Animals	Man	Sexual	Asexual
Saprobic (geophilic)	+	−	−	+	+
Saprobic, occasionally pathogenic	+	∓	∓	+	+
Pathogenic for animals (zoophilic)	∓	+	+	±	+
Pathogenic for man (anthropophilic)	−	−	+	−	±

∓ = rarely; ± = some species only

4.2.2 Total dependence: commensalism

Candidiasis (Table 1) is caused by the yeast *Candida albicans*, which resembles the dermatophytes in being entirely dependent on the living host for its existence, but differs from them as to how. This fungus is a normal commensal of the human digestive tract, including the mouth, where it lives in balance with the bacterial flora. There are widely differing estimates of the proportion of the human population carrying *Candida albicans* but the figure is at least 30%. The yeast is regularly voided with the faeces and can often be found as a contaminant of the skin of the perianal and perineal regions. From such sites, and from the mouth, it is not difficult to imagine how it may be transferred to any area of healthy skin or to eating utensils and survive there for a while, perhaps for long enough to be transferred to and colonize the digestive tract of another host.

Thus cross-infection with *Candida albicans* usually results only in the setting up of a commensal relationship with the new host, not in overt disease. This weak pathogen is kept in check by the normal defence systems of the body and by competition from the bacterial flora of the gut. It can only take on a pathogenic role if some change in the circumstances of the host lowers its defences or depletes the gut flora, when endogenous infection from the patient's own internal reservoir of the fungus may set in. The few instances where cross-infection from another host heralds the immediate onset of candidiasis include the well-known 'thrush' of the mouth in infants (Fig. 4–3) which follows delivery through an infected birth canal, and some cases of venereal spread of vaginal thrush.

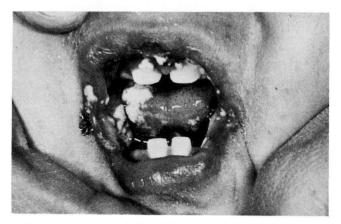

Fig. 4–3   Oral thrush in a child, caused by *Candida albicans*.

5 The Pathogenic Phase: Interaction of Host and Fungus

5.1 Preconditions for fungal invasion

Even when a fungus reaches the host it can invade only if conditions are right. As we have seen, the secondary pathogens are powerless to tackle a healthy host, but many individuals are resistant even to primary pathogens. Such people have a so-called 'natural resistance', the cause of which is unknown. For instance, it is unlikely that anyone using swimming baths or sports changing-rooms escapes contact with the fungi causing **tinea pedis** (athlete's foot) at any visit to these establishments. Yet some regular users never contract the disease and others may use the facilities for months before doing so. When attempts have been made to infect volunteers experimentally this resistance has sometimes been so marked that workers have been led to pronounce that tinea pedis is not an infectious disease.

If experimental infection in animals is a guide to events in man, the size of the fungal inoculum is critical for the establishment of many mycoses. 10^4–10^6 cells of *Candida albicans* by intravenus injection are required to kill a mouse and, again in mice, the severity of lung lesions due to *Aspergillus fumigatus* increases with the number of spores injected into the trachea: very severe lesions are induced by 13×10^7 spores. The arthrospores of *Coccidioides immitis* are far more pathogenic, for monkeys need to inhale only 10 spores and dogs 100 for an infection to be set up.

5.2 Host defences

5.2.1 Normal body defences

When a propagule of a potentially pathogenic fungus comes into contact with the human body it must, like any other microorganism, run the gauntlet of the whole armoury of the body's defences before invasion can occur. The dermatophytes can, in suitable circumstances, breach the first barrier, the skin, but other fungi must depend on introduction through a wound before they can set up a subcutaneous infection. Others again, those causing systemic mycoses, bypass the skin altogether and enter through the respiratory tract. But first they must find their way past the cilia and mucus that line this tract, and avoid the macrophages of the alveoli. If they succeed in clearing these first hurdles they will elicit to varying degrees the host's inflammatory response, antibody production and cell-mediated immunity. And in addition to all this they will have to adapt abruptly to a different (usually higher) ambient temperature and to very different sources of nutrient from those to which they had been accustomed as saprobes. For some fungi, survival in these novel conditions is marked by profound morphological change in the pathogenic phase – dimorphism – while others induce reactions in the host which result in the temporary or permanent walling off of the invaders, so delaying the progress of infection. Others again, particularly the occasional pathogens, show little visible adaptation to pathogenicity: perhaps their inability to change is the reason for their being only weak and occasional pathogens.

Candida albicans, being a human commensal in its saprobic phase, must have considerable advantages when making the change to pathogenicity. Not only is it strategically placed to colonize immediately any site in which the normal resistance is even temporarily lowered, but it is also at least partly acclimatized to any environment it will encounter as a pathogen.

5.2.2   *Barriers laid down by the host*

In many cases of lung infection the fungus is killed by the host's defences very soon after it becomes established, leaving small scars and calcifications but no living pathogen. This occurs commonly in coccidioidomycosis. In other cases the fungus may be contained by various mechanisms but is not killed so that, if the host's resistance is subsequently lowered, the dormant fungus may become reactivated and set up a secondary infection.

The **aspergilloma**, or fungal ball, is a common form of pulmonary aspergillosis. It consists of a large mass of mycelium of *Aspergillus fumigatus* filling a cavity left in the lung by another disease such as tuberculosis (Fig. 5–1). But the fungus exists there purely as a saprobe, for it is prevented from invading the surrounding tissue by a thick wall of fibrous tissue lining the cavity and laid down by the host. Only if the host subsequently becomes severely debilitated for any reason can the reactivated fungus break through the fibrous wall and invade the adjacent tissue.

When spores of *Cryptococcus neoformans* are inhaled the lesions they cause in the lungs are small and insignificant: the characteristic and damaging disease of the central nervous system is the result of blood-borne spread of the fungus from these primary lesions. Such dissemination may occur immediately after infection (primary cryptococcosis); but the lung lesions, though they do not become calcified or encapsulated, may remain in a quiescent state for many years, until some interference with the patient's immune defences results in reactivation of the fungus and the belated onset of brain lesions long after the original exposure (secondary cryptococcosis).

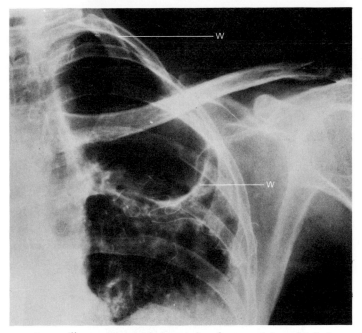

Fig. 5–1   Aspergilloma. X-ray photograph of upper lobe of left lung after surgical removal of an aspergilloma. The fibrous wall (w) round the egg-shaped cavity which remains is clearly seen.

5.3   Host/fungus products as barriers

5.3.1   Antigen-antibody precipitates

As happens with all invading organisms, fungal antigens stimulate the formation by the host of complementary protective antibodies. These antibodies can be detected in the laboratory by well-known tests in which the patient's serum is allowed to react with extracts of the fungus in conditions in which a visible precipitate is formed. Such antigen-antibody precipitates may also occur around the fungal elements in the host tissue, when they presumably help to contain the fungus and prevent its further spread through the host. *Sporothrix schenckii* furnishes a striking example of this. In its pathogenic phase this organism is a yeast and the yeast cells in the subcutaneous tissue are embedded in an amorphous, radiate substance, the antigen-antibody precipitate, to form the **asteroids** (Fig. 5–3b) which are characteristic of sporotrichosis. A similar reaction occasionally occurs with *Candida albicans* and *Aspergillus fumigatus*.

5.3.2   Biochemical reactions

Mycetoma may be caused by a wide variety of fungi, but all occur as discrete **grains** in the subcutaneous tissues and pus: only the colour, size and shape of the grains vary from fungus to fungus. Each grain consists of a colony of the fungus the outer hyphae of which are embedded in a thick layer of a hard, cement-like substance which presumably both hinders the further proliferation of the organism and protects it from the host's immunological defences (Fig. 5–2). The nature of this substance has been investigated for one of the mycetoma fungi, *Madurella mycetomatis* (FINDLAY and VISMER, 1974). In culture the fungus produces a dark, melanoid pigment which is chemically a tannin, and it was found that if a piece of collagen from a rat's tail was laid on the agar beside a colony of *Madurella mycetomatis* the pigment tanned it and transformed it into a black cement very similar to that coating a grain. Presumably this is the reaction that takes place between the fungal pigment and the host tissue proteins to form the wall of a grain.

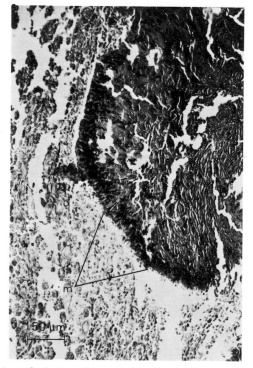

Fig. 5–2   Section of a lesion of mycetoma with a grain of *Madurella mycetomatis*. Dark-stained hyphae (m) are embedded in the wall of the grain. Periodic acid-Schiff.

5.4   Fungal response to host

5.4.1   *Dimorphism*

The morphology of the pathogenic, or tissue, phase of some fungi is conspicuously different from that of the saprobic phase, a phenomenon known as **dimorphism**. The most common change is from a mycelial mould when the fungus grows as a saprobe, to a yeast in human tissue, a change which can usually be induced in culture by eliminating sugars from the medium and incubating at body temperature. *Sporothrix schenckii* behaves in this way (Fig. 5–3), as do the fungi causing histoplasmosis, blastomycosis, and paracoccidioidomycosis (Table 2). The change in *Coccidioides immitis* is to large round spherules (see § 6.4; Fig. 6–5) which contain numerous small endospores, and this conversion too can be brought about in special cultural conditions at high temperatures. *Candida albicans* is a yeast in its commensal state but predominantly or entirely mycelial in its invasive phase (Fig. 5–4). In culture both forms frequently co-exist but manipulation of the environment can induce the dominance of one.

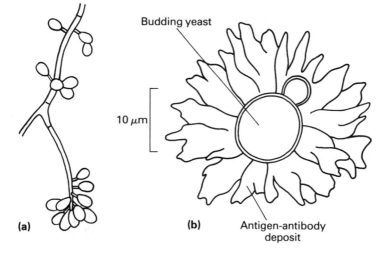

Budding yeast

10 μm

(a)   (b)   Antigen-antibody
deposit

Fig. 5–3   Dimorphism in *Sporothrix schenckii*. (a) Saprobic phase; mycelium and conidia. (b) Tissue phase; section of an asteroid showing yeast form.

5.4.2   *Dermatophyte response*

The complexity of the saprobic growth form of the dermatophytes is very much reduced by pathogenicity. Macro- and microconidia are suppressed and the fungi grow simply as sterile hyphae which, occasionally in skin and nail and always on hairs break up into arthrospores (Fig. 7–2). The perforating organs by means of which these fungi attack hard keratin in the saprobic phase (Fig. 4–1) are never found *in vivo* and fronded mycelium is formed only in nails.

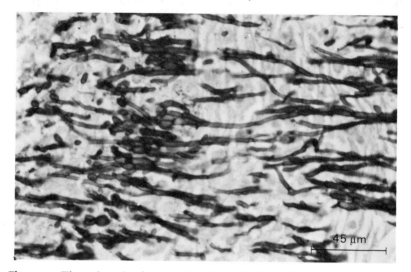

45 µm

Fig. 5–4   Tissue invasion by *Candida albicans*. Section of an oesophageal lesion showing the mycelial, invasive form of the fungus. Grocott silver stain.

6 Some Mycoses I. Occasional Pathogens: Systemic Infections and their Treatment

6.1 Mycoses due to occasional pathogens

Fungi causing these infections are pre-eminently opportunists. The onset of an infection depends on the unlikely chance of a saprobic fungus coming into contact with a host in an abnormally receptive state which the organism happens to be equipped to exploit. A remarkable instance is the single reported case of infection of the heart by a toadstool-producing fungus, *Coprinus cinereus*, one of the Ink Cap group. The asexual spores gained entry to this normally sheltered site during an 'open heart' operation, an unusual event in itself, but by a further unlucky chance *C. cinereus* is one of the very few toadstools capable of growth at the temperature of the human body. It is much more common to find these occasional pathogens affecting sites which are already exposed, such as the ear canal (otomycosis), an injured cornea (keratomycosis) and damaged nails (onychomycosis).

The morphology of occasional pathogens is very rarely modified in the pathogenic phase and they may even sporulate as if growing in culture (Fig. 6–1). Correct diagnosis depends on the alertness of the mycologist.

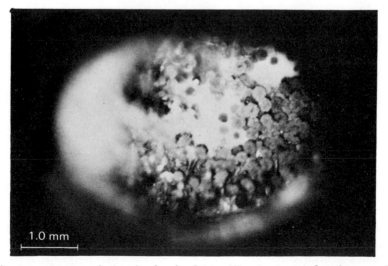

1.0 mm

Fig. 6–1 Otomycosis. Sporing heads of *Aspergillus niger* in an infected ear canal.

Not only must he be able to identify a wide range of saprobic fungi, but he must also distinguish between their presence as pathogens and as mere contaminants of his cultures.

6.2   Pulmonary aspergillosis

As a saprobe *Aspergillus fumigatus* is a fast-growing mould that thrives at the high temperatures of the rotting vegetable matter on which it lives. It produces enormous numbers of air-dispersed conidia on its mop-like sporing heads (Fig. 6–2) (an **aspergillum** is a mop for distributing holy water). These conidia are ubiquitous in the air of town and country alike, and they can give rise to pulmonary aspergillosis if inhaled. But *A. fumigatus* is a secondary pathogen which can neither invade nor colonize healthy lungs. It can only affect persons whose lungs are already damaged by some other, primary disease and even then, in the great majority of cases, its behaviour is that of a saprobe, not a pathogen. The two most common forms of pulmonary aspergillosis are the aspergilloma and allergic aspergillosis. Which form develops in a given patient will be determined by the nature of that patient's primary lung condition, but in neither form is the fungus normally invasive.

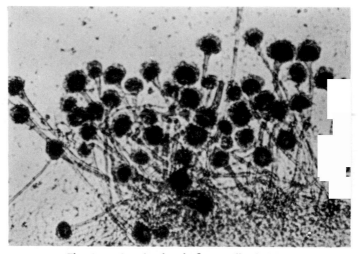

Fig. 6–2   Sporing head of *Aspergillus fumigatus*.

The **aspergilloma**, or fungus ball, in which the fungus colonizes old tuberculous and other cavities, has already been described (see § 5.2 ; Fig. 5–1). In most cases it is benign but, if following deterioration in the patient's general condition, treatment becomes necessary, the fungal mass is removed at operation.

Allergic aspergillosis (see also § 9.4) Both the spores and mycelium of *Aspergillus fumigatus* may act as allergens in atopic persons (those subject to asthma, hay fever, etc.). When the spores are inhaled by such people they are retained on the bronchial surface and may then germinate in the lumen of the bronchus to form tough plugs of mycelium embedded in mucus (Fig. 6–3a). But, as in an aspergilloma, the fungus remains a saprobe and does not invade the tissues. The allergic reaction that is set up in the adjacent bronchial wall exacerbates the patient's underlying asthmatic state and in addition the mucoid plugs may block the bronchi. At present there is no satisfactory therapy for allergic aspergillosis, but treatment of the asthmatic state gives the patient prompt relief.

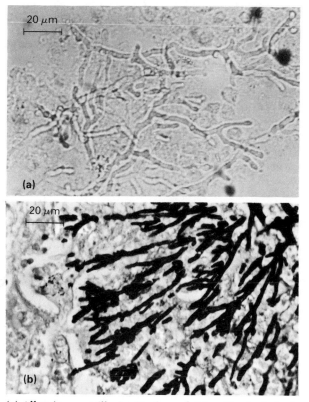

Fig. 6–3 (a) Allergic aspergillosis. Hyphae of *Aspergillus fumigatus* in a sputum plug. KOH squash preparation. (b) Invasive aspergillosis. Colony of *Aspergillus fumigatus* invading lung tissue. Grocott silver stain.

Invasive aspergillosis Only in patients already gravely ill with some major disease, particularly those under treatment with cortisone-derived **steroids** or with immunosuppressive drugs, both of which interfere with the body's natural immune defences, can *Aspergillus fumigatus* actively invade the tissue (Fig. 6–3b), an event which usually heralds death. Once tissue invasion starts it proceeds very rapidly and a diagnosis of invasive aspergillosis is often made only at the post mortem examination. Even if the disease is diagnosed in life, attempts at treatment are rarely successful.

6.3   Cryptococcosis

In culture *Cryptococcosis neoformans* is a capsulated yeast, and it has always been assumed that this is also the form in which it grows wild and is dispersed from the pigeon droppings which are its usual habitat. However, the sexual spores (basidiospores) of this fungus have recently been discovered (KWON-CHUNG, 1975). They are produced in long chains and could be the infective agents. *C. neoformans* is not a pigeon pathogen, nor a normal inhabitant of the bird's digestive tract; it merely shows a preference for their droppings as a substrate in its saprobic phase. In man, inhalation of propagules of the fungus scattered by disturbance of the dried droppings results in primary lung lesions which are usually insignificant and heal rapidly; it is as a disease of the central nervous system, following haematogenous spread from the lung, that cryptococcosis typically manifests itself (see § 5.2).

In the brain *Cryptococcus neoformans* is found in large colonies in which the small yeast cells are embedded in enormous masses of gelatinous

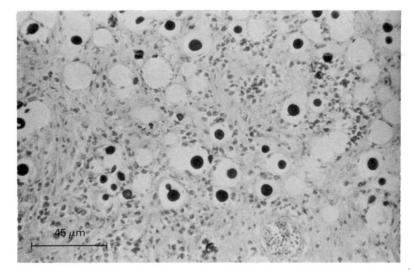

Fig. 6–4   *Cryptococcus neoformans* in brain tissue. Budding yeast cells (black) surrounded by wide (unstained) capsules. Mucicarmine.

capsular material (Fig. 6–4). The fungus can usually be demonstrated, too, in the cerebrospinal fluid, providing a sure method of diagnosis. Serological diagnostic methods are not very satisfactory in cryptococcosis. The symptoms and signs of the disease are those of meningitis. Patients who are not already mortally ill with some other primary disease may respond to drug therapy (see below).

6.4   Coccidioidomycosis

The saprobic phase of the dimorphic fungus *Coccidioides immitis*, which grows in desert soil in the American continent, produces thick-walled, air-dispersed spores which both enable the fungus to survive in the extreme soil conditions of its habitat, and are the source of infection in coccidioidomycosis (see § 3.4; Fig. 6–5a). In the lung these spores transform directly into the large, thick-walled **spherules** (Fig. 6–5b) which form the pathogenic phase. The spherules contain numerous small **endospores** which are liberated into the tissue and can form new foci of infection. Coccidioidomycosis is nearly always a minor, self-limiting disease of the lungs from which residents in endemic areas recover spontaneously, and this primary infection confers permanent immunity to further infection. Persons resident outside an endemic area have no such resistance and may contract coccidioidomycosis on entry. Occasionally the mild primary disease may progress to a severe, disseminated form which can be fatal despite treatment.

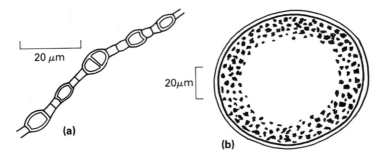

Fig. 6–5 *Coccidioides immitis.* (a) Saprobic phase; chains of thick-walled spores. (b) Tissue phase; spherule with cytoplasmic contents dividing into endospores.

It was not until some years after the discovery, at the turn of the century, of the cause of this rare, disseminated form of coccidioidomycosis, that the much more common, mild, self-limiting type was described. Knowledge of its existence, and of the geographic areas to which *Coccidioides immitis* is limited, is very largely due to extensive immunological studies on local populations. Patients who have recovered from even the mildest form of coccidioidomycosis give a positive reaction to a skin test with an extract of *C. immitis*. Therefore by testing a representative sample of the population, not only was it possible to estimate the proportion which had had the disease, but the boundaries of the area to which the fungus is indigenous were also defined.

6.5   Drug therapy of systemic mycoses

Drugs available for the treatment of systemic mycoses are far from satisfactory but some facts about those at present in use are given here.

Amphotericin B is a polyene antibiotic obtained from the actinomycete *Streptomyces nodosus*. It damages the fungal cell by binding to the sterols of the cell membrane, allowing potassium and other essential components of the cytoplasm to leak out. Most fungi are sensitive to it, but it must be given intravenously and may have serious side effects.

5-Fluorocytosine is a fluorinated pyrimidine which interferes with the pyrimidine metabolism of the fungal cell. It is given by mouth and has few side effects, but only certain fungi, notably *Candida albicans* and *Cryptococcus neoformans*, are sensitive to it, and it has the serious disadvantage that the organisms may develop resistance during treatment.

The **imidazoles** are a recently discovered group of drugs which act by increasing the permeability of the cell membrane. Most fungi are sensitive to them and they may be given by mouth or intravenously. They have not been in use for long but show considerable promise.

7 Some Mycoses II. Subcutaneous and Cutaneous Infections: Candidiasis

7.1 Mycetoma (maduromycosis)

Mycetoma can be caused by aerobic and anaerobic actinomycetes as well as by a variety of fungi, but whatever the causal organism the signs are the same; hard, nodular swellings form in the limb and from these swellings emerge sinuses (channels) which discharge pus containing 'grains' of that organism. Here we shall consider only **eumycetoma**, that is, mycetoma caused by fungi.

The list of fungi capable of causing this condition is a long one but *Petriellidium boydii, Madurella mycetomatis* and *Madurella grisea* are probably the most common, the species found depending to some extent on climatic conditions (see § 3.5). Development of lesions (Fig. 7–1a) follows minor trauma of the skin by an object infected with the fungus, and the fungal grains (see § 5.3; Fig. 7–1b) may be found both in the tissue and in the pus. Progress of the lesion along the limb is slow but

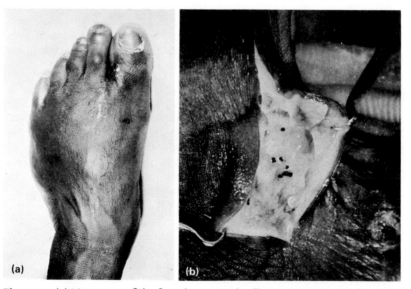

(a)   (b)

Fig. 7–1 (a) Mycetoma of the foot due to *Madurella grisea* in a West Indian. The exploratory incision (b) was made near the base of the big toe and the dark grains of the fungus were found in the subcutaneous tissue.

remorseless and at present the only treatment available for eumycetoma is excision of the lesion in very early cases, or amputation of the limb in the more advanced cases usually seen. **Actinomycetoma** (mycetoma caused by Actinomycetes) usually, however, responds well to antibacterial antibiotics, so correct identification of the causal organism is of vital importance in this disease.

7.2   Sporotrichosis

Like mycetoma, sporotrichosis is usually a wound infection, but there is only one causal organism, the mould *Sporothrix schenckii* (Fig. 5–3a), which grows on timber and plant surfaces in many parts of the world. The largest recorded outbreak of sporotrichosis was in South Africa in 1947, when over 3000 African gold miners contracted the disease. *S. schenckii* was found growing prolifically on the wooden pit props used in the mines and inoculation was occurring through minor cuts and abrasions sustained by the men in the course of their work. Because the environment in which the outbreak occurred was both man-made and totally isolated from the natural world, it was possible to control it by treating the pit props with a fungicide. In the more common small outbreaks and single cases of sporotrichosis contracted from natural environments, it is often difficult to trace the source of the fungus and therefore to control the disease.

Sporothrix schenckii is a dimorphic fungus with a yeast-like tissue phase (see § 5.4; Fig. 5–3b). The first lesion to appear is a subcutaneous abscess at the site of the wound, then further abscesses occur along the lymphatics draining the area. Sporotrichosis responds well to potassium iodide given by mouth though the mode of action of the drug is unknown.

7.3   Dermatophytosis (ringworm, tinea)

The three closely related genera of dermatophyte fungi, *Microsporum, Trichophyton* and *Epidermophyton*, can only be distinguished from one another in culture, when conidia are produced, for the morphology of the tissue phase is reduced to mycelium and arthrospores only (Fig. 7–2). In culture each genus bears distinctive multicellular macroconidia (Fig. 7–3 a–c) and in addition the genera *Microsporum* and *Trichophyton* produce unicellular microconidia (Fig. 7–3d). Dermatophytes grow only in the keratinized zones of the skin, hair and nails. In the smooth skin, growth spreads outwards to produce approximately circular, red, scaly, itchy lesions (Fig. 7–4b); in the toe-webs (tinea pedis, athlete's foot) the lesions are red, itchy and may be macerated or cracked (Fig. 7–4a); scalp lesions vary, according to the causal fungus, from diffuse loss of hair to very severe and painful lesions secondarily infected by bacteria; finger- and toe-nails become discoloured, thickened, and either very hard or flaky.

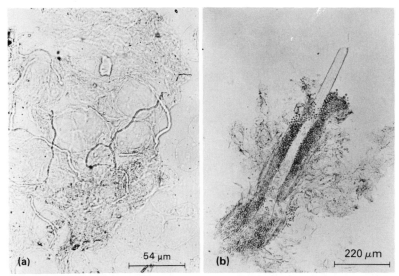

Fig. 7–2 (a) KOH squash preparation of a skin scraping containing dermatophyte hyphae; (b) KOH squash preparation showing a vellus hair infected by *Trichophyton verrucosum*. The follicle is packed with arthrospores of the fungus.

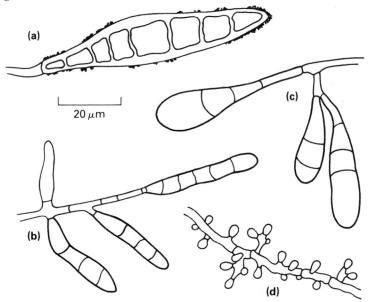

Fig. 7–3 Conidia of dermatophytes. Macroconidia of (a) *Microsporum* (b) *Trichophyton* (c) *Epidermophyton* (d) Microconidia of *Microsporum* and *Trichophyton*.

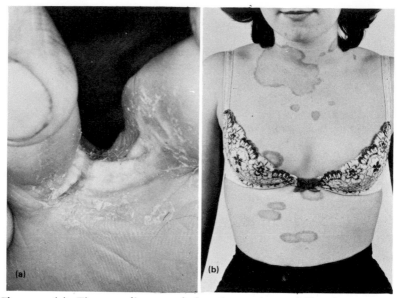

Fig. 7–4 (a) Tinea pedis caused by the anthropophilic dermatophyte *Trichophyton interdigitale*. (b) Body ringworm caused by the zoophilic dermatophyte *Trichophyton verrucosum*.

Dermatophyte species may be anthropophilic or zoophilic (see § 4.2) and infection by either type is by direct or indirect contact with an infected host for, although dermatophytes do not grow in the environment they can survive for long periods in the fragments of keratinized material in which they are shed from their host, provided these remain dry so that overgrowth by other microorganisms is prevented.

Some dermatophytes are found all over the world while others are confined to specific geographic areas. Six species are common in Britain, three anthropophilic and three zoophilic, each with its own distinctive behaviour pattern (Table 4). In Third World countries anthropophilic species causing tinea pedis are far less common than in Britain and other more affluent lands, being replaced by species causing scalp and body ringworm, diseases associated with poverty and low standards of living. In addition to the zoophilic species shown in Table 4 others are specific to horses, voles, hedgehogs, chickens and monkeys, and all of them are transferable to man.

Numerous creams and ointments are available for the treatment of tinea pedis and ringworm of the smooth skin. None is entirely effective and some are inordinately expensive. **Whitfield's ointment** (active ingredients, salicylic and benzoic acids) is as good as any, and is cheap. Scalp and nail infections, and severe or extensive infections of the skin, especially those caused by *Trichophyton rubrum*, are treated with the antifungal antibiotic **griseofulvin**, given by mouth. This drug is obtained from the mould *Penicillium griseofulvum* and is a fungistatic substance which causes curling and stunting of the hyphae of certain fungi, including the dermatophytes. In man it is adsorbed on to newly forming keratin rendering it resistant to infection, but the drug does not penetrate mature keratin or affect the hyphae already established in it. Consequently treatment must be continued until all the infected keratinized tissue has grown out, which may take a year or more in the case of toe-nails.

Table 4 Some common British dermatophytes.

Fungus	Source	Usual infection sites
Anthropophilic species		
Tricophyton interdigitale	Communal bathing places	Feet and toe-nails
Trichophyton rubrum	Family; communal bathing places	Feet and toe-nails spreading to hands, groin, etc.
Epidermophyton floccosum	Shared towels, etc., communal bathing places	Groin, feet
Zoophilic species		
Microsporum canis	Cats, dogs	Scalp (children), trunk, arms, face
Tricophyton verrucosum	Cattle	Trunk, arms, face, scalp
Tricophyton mentagrophytes	Rodents: wild, tame, laboratory	Trunk, arms, face

7.4 Candidiasis (candidosis)

Candida albicans, as a normal commensal of the human gut (see § 4.2), is a classic opportunistic pathogen, well placed to take advantage of a temporary or permanent lowering of resistance in any organ of the host's body. It is an extraordinarily versatile organism and some of the varied types of disease which it can induce, together with their precipitating causes, are listed in Table 5. Many cases of candidiasis, including some skin infections and thrush and most systemic infections, are **iatrogenic** (induced by medical procedures) and follow the use of steroids, broad-spectrum antibacterial antibiotics and immunosuppressive drugs, catheterization, and certain operations. Chronic mucocutaneous candidiasis, however, is a result of congenital deficiencies in the immune system, or sometimes in iron absorption. In this recently recognized

Table 5   Some types of candidiasis.

Clinical type	Predisposing factors/source
Oral thrush (babies) (Fig. 4–3)	Birth infection from mother
Oral thrush (adults)	Ill-fitting dentures, debility, immunosuppressive drugs
Vaginal thrush	Pregnancy, the Pill, sexual partner
Infection of body folds	Uncontrolled diabetes, steroids
Chronic paronychia (nail-fold infection)	Wet work (housewives, barmaids, etc.)
Systemic candidiasis (various organs)	Immunosuppressive drugs, steroids, antibacterial antibiotics, surgical procedures, drug addiction (via dirty needles)
Chronic mucocutaneous candidiasis	Congenital immunodeficiencies: poor iron absorption
Keratomycosis (corneal infection)	Trauma, steroids

condition severe and chronic oral thrush in childhood is followed by generalized candidiasis, especially the development of horny excrescences on the face, scalp, finger- and toe-nails.

The laboratory diagnosis of any form of candidiasis is complicated by the status of *Candida albicans* as a normal member of the gut flora, for when the fungus is isolated from a pathological specimen it is often difficult to be sure whether it is the sought-for pathogen or a mere contaminant. But direct microscopy of the original specimen can give valuable clues. If large quantities of the mycelial (tissue) phase are seen (Fig. 5–4) the likelihood of pathogenicity is far greater than if only small quantities of the yeast (commensal) phase are present. Both the methods in common use for distinguishing *C. albicans* from the many non-pathogenic yeasts isolated in medical laboratories depend on the ease with which it converts to the mycelial form. Growth on low nutrient media under micro-aerophilic conditions encourages the formation of mycelium in all species of *Candida*, but the large, terminal chlamydospores produced by *C. albicans* under these conditions are unique (Fig. 7–5). In the serum–germ-tube test the yeast to be identified is incubated for 2 hours at 37°C in horse or human serum. *C. albicans* germinates by means of germ tubes but all other species bud in the usual way.

Thrush and skin infections are treated with applications of nystatin, a polyene related to Amphotericin B, with Amphotericin B itself and with the imidazoles, and treatment for deep-seated conditions is similar to that for cryptococcosis. In mucocutaneous candidiasis treatment is aimed first at correcting the underlying defects of the immune or iron-absorption systems.

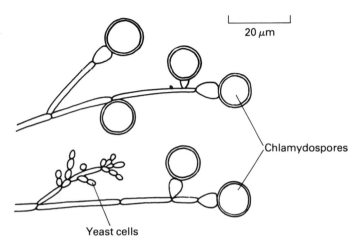

Fig. 7–5 *Candida albicans* in culture. Terminal chlamydospores formed under micro-aerophilic conditions.

8 The Pattern of Fungal Infection

8.1 Gaps in the record

Meaningful discussion of the pattern of fungal disease should assume a reasonably accurate knowledge of the distribution of the various mycoses in different parts of the world. But though such information has increased enormously in recent years it is still, for various reasons, far from complete. For instance, allergic aspergillosis is difficult to distinguish from asthma unless a deliberate search is made for it. But even if it is diagnosed there is no specific treatment, consequently the search is seldom made, and there can be little doubt that the incidence of the disease is seriously underestimated.

The gross shortage of medical facilities in vast areas of the Third World must also result in inaccurate estimates of the incidence of fungal disease in these areas. The situation referred to by AJELLO (1970) as the 'medical mycological iceberg' prevails in such places, and only the tip of the iceberg, in terms of the recorded numbers of cases, has as yet been glimpsed. However, we know already that many primary mycoses which are rare or non-existent in developed countries occur commonly in many less fortunate nations, and that they are often needlessly crippling, disfiguring or even fatal because of lack of medical attention in the early stages.

In recent years modern diagnostic techniques, especially serology, have greatly improved our knowledge of the prevalence of mycoses such as coccidioidomycosis, in which the great majority of patients may have few or no clinical signs of disease. Histoplasmosis (Table 2) is another such mycosis. Until recently it was thought to occur only in the Americas, but programmes of skin testing with histoplasmin (an extract of the causal fungus, *Histoplasma capsulatum*) have now detected sensitivity in many other parts of the world. The incidence of other systemic mycoses awaits investigation in like manner.

Despite such obvious gaps in our knowledge, there is now a sufficient body of information about the epidemiology of the mycoses for an enquiry into the pattern of their incidence to be of value.

8.2 Factors governing the distribution of mycoses

The occurrence of a particular mycosis in a particular locality depends on three things – the ability of the causal fungus to complete its life cycle there, whether it is primarily a saprobe, an obligate parasite or a commensal; the availability of dispersal routes allowing its passage to fresh hosts; and a low threshold of resistance in an appreciable number of the local population. Clearly a disease cannot occur where its causal fungus is unable, for whatever reason, to survive. But this is less of a limiting factor than might be supposed for, as we have seen, many human pathogens are cosmopolitan or, if they are not, the same clinical disease can be caused by another fungus in another locality, e.g. ringworm, mycetoma. In general the resistance of the host probably more often limits the incidence of a mycosis than does the absence of the fungus.

8.3   Distribution of primary mycoses caused by saprobes

Because these diseases can only be contracted following exposure to the saprobic phase of the fungus their prevalence is controlled in the first place by environmental factors affecting that phase. The reasons for the limited geographical range of coccidioidomycosis have already been discussed (see § 3.4). The saprobic phase of *Histoplasma capsulatum* (Fig. 8–1) also has specific requirements, for though the fungus is found in most parts of the world it grows only in districts in which the soils are enriched by bird or bat droppings. Histoplasmosis occurs in persons who have recently cleaned out old fowl houses, disturbed the droppings under the roosting sites of wild birds, or who have visited caves and other places where bats congregate. As is the case with coccidioidomycosis, skin tests show that up to 90% of those exposed to infected soils may have had a mild form of the disease. And again as in coccidioidomycosis this mild form may occasionally progress to a disseminated and fatal form.

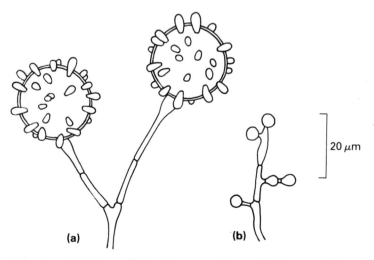

Fig. 8–1   Saprobic phase of *Histoplasma capsulatum*. (a) Macroconidia and (b) Microconidia.

In both coccidioidomycosis and histoplasmosis attempts have been made to discover whether there is any special factor predisposing to the disseminated forms of the diseases. None has been found for histoplasmosis. But in coccidioidomycosis males are four times more likely to progress to this form than females, and coloured races are from three to 175 times more likely to succumb to it than whites. It is improbable, however, that differences in either racial or sexual susceptibility are directly responsible for this. The explanation would seem to lie in the poverty and consequent malnutrition, and the inadequate medical attention, that are the lot of the coloured races in coccidioidomycosis areas and, especially for males, in their long hours of work on the land and consequent massive exposure to the spores of *Coccidioides immitis*.

Blastomycosis and paracoccidioidomycosis (Table 2) are also overwhelmingly diseases of the underprivileged, but comparatively little is known as yet of their epidemiology.

Among the subcutaneous mycoses not only mycetoma and sporotrichosis, but chromomycosis and phycomycosis (Table 2) are primarily diseases of the Third World and the underprivileged. It is not simply that the causal fungi flourish best in warm climates, for many are known in temperate regions. But the way of life of the people, adults and children alike, brings them into constant and close contact with the soil and its vegetation, they wear few or no clothes, and any slight scratch or graze of the unprotected skin can lead to inoculation with a pathogenic fungus. Subcutaneous phycomycosis is predominantly a disease of childhood caused by a member of the Zygomycotina, *Basidiobolus ranarum*. This fungus is found in the soil, on decaying vegetation and also in the intestinal tracts of frogs, and would gain entry to the host through minor wounds and abrasions incurred as the scantily clad children play in any available space in and around their villages. More hygienic playgrounds for children, and protective footwear for adults, would reduce the incidence of the subcutaneous mycoses dramatically and they should almost disappear with improving standards of living.

In summary, the primary mycoses caused by a saprobic fungi, at least in their severe forms and with the exception of histoplasmosis, are overwhelmingly diseases of deprived races and communities in which exposure to the causal fungi may be intense, host resistance is low through malnutrition, and medical aid inadequate.

8.4   Distribution of secondary infections by opportunistic fungi

Candida albicans, Aspergillus fumigatus and *Cryptococcus neoformans*, together with *Mucor* and *Absidia* spp. causing systemic phycomycosis (Figs 1–1, 1–2a) (Table 2), are the fungi responsible for by far the largest number of secondary mycoses, and all, like their preferred habitats –

namely man himself, decaying vegetable matter and pigeon droppings respectively – are of world-wide distribution. There is little likelihood that any human being escapes contact with them at one time or another. Yet candidiasis, aspergillosis, secondary cryptococcosis (as distinct from the primary form) and systemic phycomycosis are very rarely seen in Third World countries or in deprived communities in more advanced countries, despite the low resistance of these people to the primary mycoses. On the contrary, the secondary mycoses are pre-eminently diseases of affluence and are causing increasing problems in technologically advanced countries. For it is only in these countries that patients with debilitating or mortal illnesses such as diabetes, heart and kidney conditions, various forms of cancer and certain congenital diseases, are submitted to sophisticated medical and surgical procedures which, either as an unintentional side effect, or deliberately in the case of transplant surgery, reduce or almost eliminate the immunological defences. These same procedures then keep the patient alive for long enough to permit invasion by such extremely weak pathogens as the opportunistic fungi.

The circumstances predisposing to candidiasis and cryptococcosis have already been discussed (see § 7.4 and § 5.2) and include debility from pre-existing grave disease, often aggravated by the use of antibacterial antibiotics, steroids and immunosuppressant drugs in the treatment of that disease. Pulmonary aspergillosis has been shown to be secondary to various unrelated lung conditions, but *Aspergillus fumigatus* is more than a pulmonary pathogen for in suitable circumstances it can invade almost any part of the body to which it can gain entry. It is troublesome in both open heart and transplant operations – the death of Britain's first heart transplant patient was at least partly attributable to secondary infection by *A. fumigatus*. The fungus can also infect the ears, eyes and nasal sinuses, and may be associated with thrombi, though whether it induces these by blocking blood vessels, or merely colonizes an existing thrombus is unknown.

To summarize, infections by opportunistic fungi are diseases of populations whose economic well-being ensures them excellent basic health, good working conditions and adequate medical attention. These confer resistance to primary fungal pathogens and permit survival of other hitherto fatal diseases, but only at the risk of the patient eventually falling victim to an opportunistic fungus, the weakest pathogen of all.

8.5   Distribution of the dermatophytoses

The prevalence of this group of diseases, caused by fungi with no saprobic or commensal phase, is entirely determined by the way of life of the host, for this governs not only the condition of the substrate – the human body – but the means of spread available to the fungus.

Ringworm due to zoophilic dermatophytes is commonly an occupational hazard, especially of farm workers, and the species of fungus causing the infection will depend on the animal contacts of the worker. For instance, in Czechoslovakia it has been shown that *Trichophyton verrucosum* is the usual cause of human ringworm in the large, modern dairy farms in the south of the country, but that peasant farmers in the mountainous north are usually infected by *Trichophyton mentagrophytes* which they catch from the wild rodents infesting their barns.

Each of the anthropophilic dermatophytes has its own predilection for specific sites on the human body. We have seen that the three species found most commonly in Britain are primarily foot or groin pathogens, though *Trichophyton rubrum* may spread to other sites later. None of them causes scalp ringworm or primary body ringworm, and these diseases are rare in Britain as in all well-to-do countries and communities. Tinea pedis is a comparatively recent affliction of man which only came into existence in the late nineteenth century but has spread with incredible rapidity since, to become today the most common form of ringworm in the developed countries (Fig. 8–2). Its success seems to be due equally to the universal wearing of shoes and hose, which ensure an excellent substrate for the fungi by keeping the feet warm and moist, and the regular use of bathrooms, swimming-baths and changing-rooms, together with the communal living conditions in boarding-schools and similar establishments, where cross-infection to healthy feet can take place readily.

In contrast to tinea pedis, scalp and body ringworm due to anthropophilic dermatophytes (as distinct from those due to zoophilic species) have been known since ancient times and are always associated with poverty. They did not die out in Britain or other now affluent countries until the first half of this century and in Japan scalp ringworm has only just been conquered. Poor hygiene, lack of medical facilities and possibly also malnutrition are responsible for their persistence, and overcrowding for their spread. These diseases will gradually be eliminated as living conditions improve but will doubtless be replaced by tinea pedis, as in the advanced countries today.

Fig. 8–2   Map showing the world distribution of tinea pedis and of scalp and body ringworm due to anthropophilic dermatophytes.

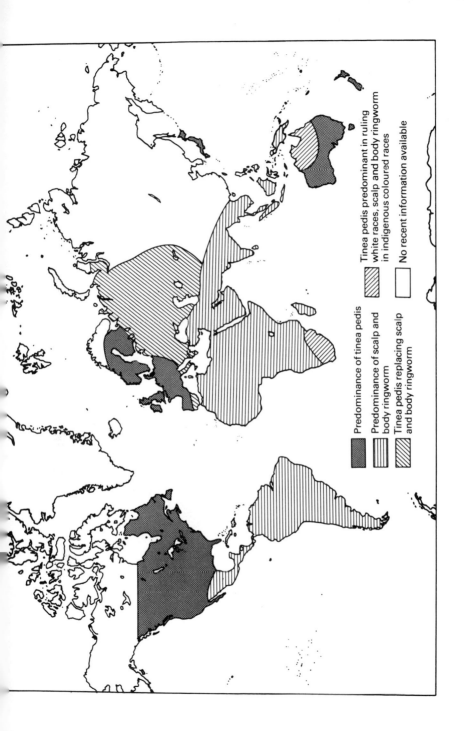

Predominance of tinea pedis

Predominance of scalp and
body ringworm

Tinea pedis replacing scalp
and body ringworm

Tinea pedis predominant in ruling
white races, scalp and body ringworm
in indigenous coloured races

No recent information available

9 Fungal Hypersensitivities

While some airborne fungal spores are, as we have seen, agents of infectious disease, others make their impact on man as allergens, and are responsible for distressing respiratory conditions if inhaled by sensitized persons. Such persons suffer from allergic disease and are said to be **hypersensitive**.

Much is known of the air spora (the spore and pollen grain content of the atmosphere) through the studies both of allergists and of plant pathologists investigating the epidemiology of crop disease, and an excellent account of present knowledge has been given by GREGORY (1973). The Hirst spore trap, by means of which air-borne spores are impacted on to sticky glass slides (Fig. 9–1), is a most convenient method for examining the air spora. From observations made with this machine it is known that in temperate climates the fungal spores most generally abundant are those of *Alternaria* and *Cladosporium* (Fig. 1–2d and e), moulds found on dying grasses and cereals especially in late summer and autumn. Allergic reactions to these two fungi are, however, rare and it is rather to locally high concentrations of less common spores that sensitivities are usually recorded.

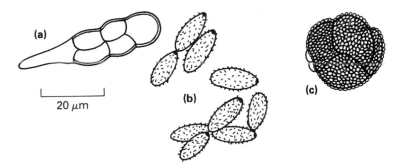

Fig. 9–1 Fungal spores impacted on a slide from a Hirst trap. (a) *Alternaria*; (b) *Cladosporium.* sp. and (c) *Epicoccum* sp.

9.1 Types of allergic reaction to fungi

Allergic reactions are the body's immunological response to many foreign materials with which it may come into contact, materials which are known collectively as **antigens**. The complex chemicals coating the surfaces of fungal spores are antigenic in nature. Contact with an antigen stimulates the body to produce complementary **antibodies** of various types which react with the antigen to neutralize it, a valuable defence mechanism in the normal course of events but the cause of serious illness if occurring in an uncontrolled way. Chemically these antibodies, known as humoral antibodies, are **immunoglobulins** (Ig) and five different types, each mediating a different type of reaction, are known. In fungal hyper-sensitivity two of these immunoglobulins have an overwhelmingly important role – IgE, produced in large quantities by atopic persons (those subject to hay fever, asthma and eczema), and IgG, the dominant antibody produced by non-atopic persons. IgE reacts with the antigen at the cell surface immediately the two substances come into contact in the skin or at a mucous membrane, and pharmacologically active substances are released. This is known as a **Type I reaction** and is detected by means of a skin test with an extract of the fungus. The response of IgG, on the other hand, does not occur until several hours after exposure to the antigen and, because the antibody circulates in the serum, the reaction takes place in tissue spaces where an antigen–antibody precipitate forms. This is a **Type III reaction**, and it can also be detected by means of a skin test, but the response to the test is slow, taking about eight hours to develop. Type III sensitivities are commonly detected by means of bench tests in which the patient's serum is allowed to precipitate against an extract of the fungus.

Because IgE and IgG antibodies act at different sites the type of illness caused by excessive production of either will differ. In atopic patients, whose illness is mediated by IgE, the hypersensitive reaction takes place in the bronchial walls against fungal material adhering to them and this results in an immediate attack of **bronchial asthma**. In non-atopic patients fungal spores lodge in the alveoli and react with IgG antibodies in the adjacent tissue spaces giving rise to **allergic alveolitis**, that is, difficulty in breathing and other symptoms which only become evident a few hours after exposure to the fungal spores. These attacks increase in severity with repeated exposure until permanent damage to the lung tissue sets in, but protection from exposure before that point is reached results in complete recovery. The two types of hypersensitivity are compared in Table 6.

9.2 Asthma and 'hay' fever due to fungi

Allergy to those fungal spores most commonly found in the atmosphere is very rare compared with that due to pollen grains. But sensitivity occasionally occurs to the spores of fungi causing disease in cultivated plants, spores which may occur in dense clouds down wind from an infected crop. *Puccinia graminis*, the cause of black rust of wheat, and the bunts and smuts of cereals caused by species of *Ustilago* and *Tilletia*, are notable examples. In market gardens glasshouse tomatoes are

Table 6   Characteristics of fungal hypersensitivity diseases.

Characteristic	Bronchial asthma (Type I hypersensitivity)	Allergic alveolitis (Type III hypersensitivity)
Allergic status of patient	Atopic	Non-atopic
Mediating antibody	IgE	IgG
Site of reaction	Cell surface	Tissue spaces
Onset of attack	Immediate	Delayed
Result of:		
skin test	Immediate wheal	Delayed swelling
bench test	—	Antigen/antibody precipitate

sometimes affected by the leaf-mould fungus *Fulvia fulva* with the result that sensitized workers, while they can enter a 'clean' glass-house with impunity, develop immediate asthmatic symptoms on entering one in which leaf-mould is present. Sensitivity to the abundantly produced spores of the dry-rot fungus, *Serpula lacrimans* (*Merulius lachrymans*), is also well known. Occasional cases of sensitivity to the spores of many named species of fungi have been reported but proof has seldom been rigorous and their authenticity is often doubtful.

9·3   Allergic alveolitis

This condition can be caused by organic dusts and by the spores of actinomycetes (e.g. farmer's lung) as well as by fungal spores, but only the latter will be considered here.

During the malting process in whisky distilleries, barley which has been steeped in water is allowed to germinate in thick layers on malting floors, and to ensure even germination maltsters are employed to rake over and turn the grain. The moisture, combined with the heat generated by germination, provide ideal growth conditions for fungi and the barley sometimes becomes heavily infected with *Aspergillus clavatus*. Maltster's lung may then be contracted if a worker becomes sensitized to the clouds of spores liberated from the fungus during the turning process.

Maple-bark stripper's lung is a similar disease found among workers in paper-mills in the U.S.A. Maple logs are commonly used in paper-making and the bark of the standing trees is often heavily infected by the mould *Cryptostroma corticale*. Men employed to strip the bark may be affected by the spores of this fungus. Suberosis, a disease of cork-workers, and cheese-washer's lung, are similar conditions caused by species of *Penicillium* (Fig. 1–2b) contaminating the cork and cheese respectively.

9.4   Allergic aspergillosis

This disease, which has already been described briefly (see § 6.2), is unique among fungal allergies in that *Aspergillus fumigatus* actually grows in the bronchi thus ensuring that the patient is continually exposed to the fungus over long periods, whereas with all other fungi the allergy is set up by recently inhaled, ungerminated spores, so that exposure is intermittent. Allergic aspergillosis occurs in atopic persons, that is, it is primarily a Type I hypersensitivity mediated by IgE antibodies which give an immediate response to a skin test with an extract of the fungus. But most patients with allergic aspergillosis also have a weak Type III reaction, that is there is a second, delayed response to the skin test and IgG antibodies can be demonstrated in the serum. This dual reaction is probably the result of the continued stimulation of the patient's immune system by the presence in the bronchi of the growing fungus.

10 Mycetism and Mycotoxicosis

The poisonous properties of certain toadstools must have been known to man through bitter experience from time immemorial, but other forms of fungal poisoning have proved much more difficult to trace to their source. St Anthony's fire, the terrifying disease that struck whole communities without warning in the Middle Ages, was not traced to ergots until the sixteenth century, and it was only in the eighteenth century that it was generally accepted that ergots were fungal in origin. That there is a connection between liver cancer and mouldy foodstuffs has only been realized in the last twenty years.

10.1 Mycetism

Although only a few species of British toadstools are poisonous and not many people in Britain are mycophagists (toadstool eaters), cases of mycetism, or toadstool poisoning, occur nearly every autumn in this country. On the Continent, where toadstools are a sought-after delicacy and are sold in the markets as well as collected for personal use, mycetism is more common. In Poland, in the autumn, television is used to instruct would-be mycophagists on the identification of edible and poisonous toadstools.

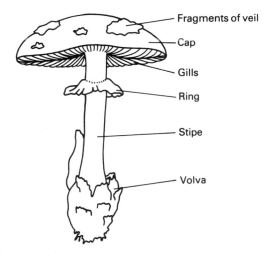

Fig. 10–1 *Amanita phalloides*, the Death Cap toadstool. The cap is pale yellowish green, streaked; gills, stipe, ring and volva are white. (After COOKE, M. C. (1894). *Edible and Poisonous Mushrooms*. S.P.C.K., London.)

The Death Cap toadstool, *Amanita phalloides* (Fig. 10–1), is by far the most common of the few deadly agarics found in this country, and is the cause of most fatalities. It grows in or at the edges of woodlands, rather than in the open pastures which are preferred by the common mushroom *Agaricus campestris*, with which it is sometimes confused. Its several toxins, the phalloidins, have a cyclic radicle (Fig. 10–2). They act primarily on the liver but also have severe effects on most other organs including the heart and kidneys.

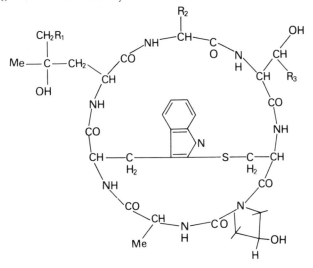

Fig. 10–2   Cyclic radicle of the phalloidin group of toxins.

Closely related to the Death Cap is the Fly Agaric, *Amanita muscaria*, with its showy red or orange cap with white spots, found in large numbers in the autumn in birch and pine woods.   Its toxins, muscimol and ibotenic acid (Fig. 10–3), are seldom fatal but the fungus can cause severe illness if eaten in excess. Despite this risk, peasants living in localities to which it is native have traditionally made use of it for its halucinogenic properties.

Though not truly toxic, the genus *Psilocybe* should perhaps be mentioned here, for a number of its members, too, have recently gained

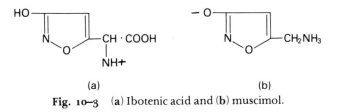

(a)   (b)

Fig. 10–3   (a) Ibotenic acid and (b) muscimol.

notoriety as hallucinogens. *Psilocybe mexicana* has been used in magic rites by Mexican peasants for centuries and still has a semi-sacred status among them today. Other less potent species, all dependent for their hallucinogenic properties on the sterols psilocin and psilocybin (Fig. 10–4), are common in Britain and Europe.

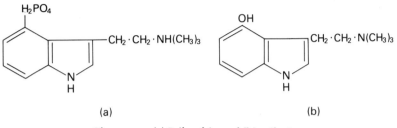

(a)   (b)

Fig. 10–4   (a) Psilocybin and (b) psilocin.

10.2   Mycotoxicosis

10.2.1   Ergotism

The ergot is the resting stage, or sclerotium, of the plant parasite *Claviceps purpurea* (Fig. 10–5). Ergots replace the seed in the flower spikes of various species of grasses but are especially common in rye. If parasitized rye is milled, the resulting flour and the bread made from it will be contaminated with the crushed ergots.

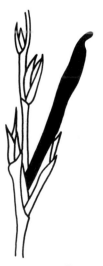

Fig. 10–5   *Claviceps purpurea*. An ergot affecting an inflorescence of rye-grass.

Over twenty potent alkaloids have been obtained from ergots, all of them with a basic structure similar to that of lysergic acid (Fig. 10–6). Purified and used in carefully controlled doses, some of them have valuable medicinal properties. But as different batches of ergot contain the alkaloids in different proportions, and as no alkaloid has the same pharmacological effect as any other, if they are eaten inadvertently and in uncontrolled doses in bread, they are potent and terrifying poisons which may result in permanent damage to health, or in death. Broadly they fall into two main pharmacological groups. Some induce constriction of the blood vessels and may be used medicinally to control haemorrhage after childbirth, but result in gangrene and necrosis of the limbs if ingested indiscriminately with the food. Others have their primary effect on the central nervous system and can be used medicinally to control migraine, but result in hallucinations, madness, convulsions and death if eaten inadvertently. In natural outbreaks of ergotism these symptoms will vary in degree and type according to the alkaloids present, the amount eaten and many other variables, thus accounting for the extraordinary differences in the characteristics of the outbreaks which were such a mystery in the medieval epidemics. Fortunately, with modern methods of food inspection, ergotism in man is now extremely rare, though there are still regular reports of outbreaks in farm animals.

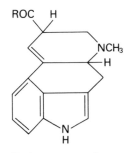

Fig. 10–6   Basic structure of an ergot alkaloid.

10.2.2   Aflatoxicosis

Moulds secrete metabolites into the substrate on which they are growing: if the metabolites are toxic to man or animals they are called mycotoxins. If bulk-stored foods and feeding-stuffs such as grain, beans or peanuts are allowed to become damp, mould infestation will set in, particularly in warm climates, and should the mould be a toxin producer those eating the product, or any foods derived from it, will run the risk of mycotoxicosis. In the last twenty or thirty years many very varied diseases of man and animals, the causes of which were previously unknown, have been shown to be due to mycotoxins of contrasting chemical composition, and work is proceeding on other diseases of mysterious origin.

Perhaps the best known and most widely investigated mycotoxin is **aflatoxin** (Fig. 10–7) produced by certain strains of *Aspergillus flavus*. Aflatoxin is a lactone, a vitamin K analogue which acts on DNA and reduces RNA synthesis. It was discovered during the investigation of two massive outbreaks of liver disease in livestock which occurred in 1960. In that year 100 000 turkey poults in Britain died of liver necrosis, and in the U.S.A. young trout in hatcheries were decimated by liver cancer. Eventually it was found that both birds and fish had been fed on mouldy groundnut meal and the origin of both types of liver disease was traced to a metabolite of *A. flavus* which was given the name aflatoxin. It is now known that a comparatively large intake of aflatoxin results in liver necrosis and speedy death, while minute doses over a long period can give rise to liver cancer, or hepatoma though some animal species, notably monkeys and mice, are scarcely affected by the toxin. In addition to its carcinogenic activities, aflatoxin is known to modify the immune system in many ways, reducing the body's resistance to invading organisms.

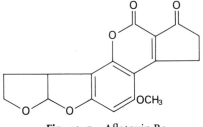

Fig. 10–7   Aflatoxin B1.

Though primary liver cancer in man is a rare disease in the developed countries it is common in the Third World, and recent epidemiological investigations have shown a clear relationship between a high frequency of the disease, a warm, damp climate suitable for mould growth, and the presence of aflatoxin in the food. But it is also known that most victims of hepatoma are chronic carriers of the hepatitis-B virus and that this virus is closely associated with predisposition to hepatoma. A recent hypothesis (LUTWICK, 1979) suggests that humans, like monkeys and mice, may be resistant to the cancer-inducing properties of aflatoxin, but that it is its action in depressing the body's immune defences that is significant in initiating hepatoma. A patient whose immune system was impaired by aflatoxin would be unable, if he became infected with hepatitis-B virus, to eliminate that virus from his body completely, and would become a chronic carrier. He would thus be subjected to long-term exposure to the hepatoma-inducing properties of the virus.

Several other human mycotoxicoses have been reported of which the most notable is probably the 'yellow rice' disease of the Far East. The mould *Penicillium islandicum* causes yellowing of stored rice grains which, if eaten, result in liver disease. The fungus produces several toxins one of which, luteoskyrin, induces cancer in laboratory animals.

11 Laboratory Diagnosis of Fungal Infection

Pathogenic fungi must be handled only under the supervision of trained personnel in properly equipped laboratories, hence practical work in medical mycology cannot be recommended to general readers of this book. This chapter merely outlines the methods of investigation that are used to diagnose mycoses in hospital laboratories.

11.1 Specimens for diagnostic mycology

Sputum and all body fluids and exudates are suitable for mycological examination. If a tissue infection by a yeast is suspected, swabbing is a satisfactory sampling method for, in addition to the mycelium within the tissue which will not be removed by swabbing, free yeast cells will be present which will be picked up. If the infecting agent is a mycelial fungus and there is a considerable amount of pus, swabbing may again be satisfactory. But if there is little or no pus the sample must consist of a fragment of the tissue. Skin scrapings, nail clippings and hairs pulled out by the roots are suitable dermatological specimens, but biopsies may be necessary for the diagnosis of deeper mycoses.

11.2 Direct microscopy and histology

Direct microscopy of tissues, sputa, etc., is extremely important in medical mycology, because so many pathogenic fungi are also common saprobes and could, if not actually seen in the specimen, be mere contaminants of the cultures in which they are found. In the invaluable potassium hydroxide squash technique, fragments of skin, hair or nails are macerated in a drop of 20% KOH on a slide, squashed under a coverslip and examined for fungal hyphae (Figs 6–3a and 7–2). This method is also useful for other tissues and for sputum.

Histological sections must be stained specifically for fungi by the periodic acid-Schiff or Grocott silver impregnation techniques (Figs 5–2 and 6–3b); haematoxylin-and-eosin is seldom of value. The Gram stain is only useful for *Candida* spp. and may be used for smears from swabs, sputum and urine provided no other fungi are suspected.

Because of the large size of fungi an oil immersion objective is not necessary in diagnostic work. An organism which is too small to be seen clearly with a × 40 objective is not a fungus.

11.3   Culture and identification of fungi

Few people working with medically important fungi have received any training in mycology, but many have some experience of bacteriology and, when confronted by a fungus, simply use bacteriological techniques to deal with it. These techniques are adequate for yeasts for, like bacteria, they are morphologically undistinguished, unicellular organisms. But it is not generally realized that bacteriological methods need considerable modification if the morphologically complex filamentous fungi are to be cultured and identified successfully and safely. In the following notes the differences between mycological and bacteriological techniques are presented and the reasons explained.

11.3.1   Cultural conditions

Media   Unlike bacteria, most fungi prefer an acid medium, pH 5–6, to an alkaline one. Sugars enhance fungal growth, glucose, sucrose and maltose being the most often used. An organic source of nitrogen is preferred to an inorganic one.

Media for isolating fungi from tissues and exudates are very simple. The best known and most generally useful is Sabouraud's agar (1% peptone, 4% glucose). This is a modification of the medium invented by the great French dermatologist who was responsible for controlling the massive outbreak of scalp ringworm among the children of Paris at the turn of the century, and who was also the first person to study the dermatophytes systematically. For fungi causing systemic and sub-cutaneous mycoses blood agar and nutrient agar, available in any hospital bacteriology laboratory, are used in addition to Sabouraud's agar. It is useful to add antibacterial antibiotics to mycological media, and the antifungal agent cyclohexamide inhibits many fungi but allows dermatophytes to grow.

Temperature   All medically important fungi grow well at 30°C, those such as *Aspergillus fumigatus* and *Candida albicans*, which grow faster at 37°C, nevertheless mature fully at the lower temperature. But most dermatophytes are severely inhibited at 37°C, and even some fungi causing deeper mycoses, *Cryptococcus neoformans* and *Madurella grisea* for example, have their optimuim temperature a few degrees below this. It is therefore advisable to incubate some cultures, at least, of all primary isolations from the patient and of any unknown fungus, at 30°C.

Aeration   Fungi are strongly aerobic, and spore production in particular is halted by an inadequate supply of oxygen. Tubes plugged with cotton-wool are preferable to screw-capped bottles as culture vessels, but if bottles are used the caps must be left loose.

Incubation time   With a few exceptions such as *Aspergillus fumigatus*, *Candida albicans* and some members of the Zygomycotina, fungi grow much more slowly than bacteria, so that it may be necessary to incubate cultures for 1–3 weeks. It follows that contamination may be a problem, and the practice of drying the surfaces of freshly poured Petri-dishes with the lids removed should be avoided.

11.3.2   Handling cultures

Many fungi have spores which are especially adapted for air dispersal and in the medical laboratory these may present serious problems of infection of personnel and contamination of other cultures if they are not correctly handled. Culture containers must not be opened unless strictly necessary, and then only for the briefest possible time. Above all, **cultures must not be smelled**.

Aerial mycelium does not adhere to bacteriological loops, neither can these loops cut through the tough submerged mycelium of a fungal colony. Stiff needles, preferably pointed, are necessary for the manipulation of fungal cultures.

11.3.3   Microscopic examination of cultures

Yeasts resemble bacteria in that nutritional tests, rather than morphology, are of prime importance in their identification. Filamentous fungi, on the other hand, are identified primarily by their infinitely varied morphological characteristics. To avoid distortion and shrinkage, wet mounts are used. The mycelium is teased out in a drop of lactophenol-cotton blue on a slide, covered with a cover-slip and examined directly. Microculture techniques, in which the fungus is grown and mounted on the slide on which it will be examined, cut down disturbance.

11.4   Fungal contaminants

It is essential that a medical mycologist should be able to identify, at least to genus level, the moulds commonly found as cultural contaminants. For not only must these be distinguished from recognized pathogens, but they may themselves become opportunistic pathogens on occasion. Most text books of medical mycology include a section on contaminants, and SMITH's 'Industrial Mycology' (1969) is invaluable for identifying both these and many occasional pathogens, especially *Aspergillus* spp. and members of the Zygomycotina. The book also has excellent sections on mycological techniques. LARONE's (1976) guide to the identification of medically important fungi also includes a selection of common contaminants.

11.5 Serological methods

In recent years serological methods, used in addition to direct microscopy and culture, have become of increasing importance in the diagnosis and monitoring of certain systemic and subcutaneous mycoses. Circulating antibodies to the invading fungus are produced by the host and can be detected in his blood serum by the standard agglutination, precipitin and immunofluorescence tests. Of the diseases discussed here, serological procedures are particularly useful in coccidioidomycosis, aspergillosis and mycetoma, but are less helpful in cryptococcosis because of the inert capsule enveloping the yeast cells, and in candidiasis because the frequent presence of the fungus as a commensal often gives false positive results.

References and Further Reading

General

EMMONS, C. W., BINFORD, C. H., UTZ, J. P. and KWON-CHUNG, K. J. (1977). *Medical Mycology*, 3rd edition. Lea and Febiger, Philadelphia. (An advanced text covering all known mycoses. Useful introductory chapters, and sections on methods and contaminants.)

Chapters 1 and 3

HUDSON, H. J. (1980). *Fungal Saprophytism*, 2nd edition. Studies in Biology, no. 32. Edward Arnold, London.
INGOLD, C. T. (1973). *The Biology of Fungi*, 2nd revised edition. Hutchinson Educational, London.

Chapter 5

FINDLAY, G. H. and VISMER, H. F. (1974). Black grain mycetoma. A study of the chemistry, formation and significance of the tissue grain in *Madurella mycetomi* infection. *Br. J. Derm.*, **91**, 297.

Chapter 6

KWON-CHUNG, K. J. (1975). Description of a new genus, *Filobasidiella*, the perfect state of *Cryptococcus neoformans*. *Mycologia*, **67**, 1197.

Chapter 8

AJELLO, L. (1970). The medical mycological iceberg. In *Proceedings International Symposium on Mycoses*. Scientific publication No. **205**, Pan American Health Organization, Washington, p. 3.
CHICK, E. W., BALOWS, A. and FURCOLOW, M. L. (Eds) (1975). Opportunistic fungal infections. *Proceedings of the Second International Conference*. Thomas, Springfield, Illinois.
ENGLISH, M. P. (1972). The epidemiology of animal ringworm in man. *Br. J. Derm.*, **86**, Suppl. 8, 78.
GENTLES, J. C., EVANS, E. G. V. and JONES, G. R. (1974). Control of tinea pedis in a swimming bath. *Br. med. J.*, **2**, 577.

Chapter 9

CHANNELL, S. *et al*. Allergic alveolitis in malt workers. *Qu. J. Med.*, **38**, 351.
GREGORY, P. H. (1973). *The Microbiology of the Atmosphere*, 2nd edition. Leonard Hill, Aylesbury.
HENDERSON, A. H. (1968). Allergic aspergillosis: review of 32 cases. *Thorax*, **23**, 501.

Chapter 10

GOLDBLATT, L. A. (Ed.) (1969). *Aflatoxin*. Academic Press, London.

LUTWICK, L. I. (1979). Relation between aflatoxin, hepatitis-B virus, and hepatocellular carcinoma. *Lancet*, Apr. 7, 755.

RAMSBOTTOM, J. (1953). *Mushrooms and Toadstools*. New Naturalist, No. 7. Collins, London. Chaps. 5, 6, 13.

Chapter 11

BENEKE, E. S. and ROGERS, A. L. (1970). *Medical Mycology Manual*, 3rd edition. Burgess, Minneapolis.

EVANS, E. G. V. (Ed.) (1976). *Serology of Fungal Infection and Farmer's Lung Disease*. British Society for Mycopathology, University of Leeds.

LARONE, D. H. (1976). *Medically Important Fungi: a Guide to Identification*. Harper and Row, San Francisco.

REBELL, G. and TAPLIN, D. (1970). *Dermatophytes, their Recognition and Identification*, 2nd edition. University of Miami Press, Florida.

SMITH, G. (1969). *An Introduction to Industrial Mycology*, 6th edition. Edward Arnold, London.

Stu

About

This is an introduction to medical mycology using
selected mycoses to illustrate the interrelationships
between fungus, host and environment, rather than
attempting a catalogue of all the major mycoses. The
diseases are grouped according to the site of the
primary infection which is found to be dependent on the
route by which the fungus enters the body. This, in turn,
depends on the method of spore dispersal in saprobic
fungi, or the route of cross-infection in obligate
pathogens and commensals. Modifications in fungal
morphology induced by the host are then discussed,
followed by descriptions of the selected diseases to
illustrate the effect on the host of the fungus. The world-
wide pattern of fungal infection in man is then
considered. Finally there are chapters on fungal
allergies, poisoning by fungi and their metabolites, and
the practical problems of handling fungi in diagnostic
laboratories.

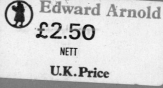

Edward Arnold
£2.50
NETT
U.K. Price

sponsored by The Institute of Biology

The series of booklets 'Studies in Biology' is sponsored by The
Institute of Biology as one of its activities in advancing the
knowledge of biology by all means and promoting the
professional standing, efficiency and usefulness of biologists.
Enquiries concerning membership of the Institute, its
privileges and facilities will be welcomed and should be
addressed to: Freepost, The Institute of Biology, 41 Queens
Gate, London, SW7 5BR.

3 1210 00343 3032

Edward Arnold (Publishers) Ltd

ISBN 0 7131 2795 3
ISSN 0537-9024